Natural Beauty Products

For Curing and Healing

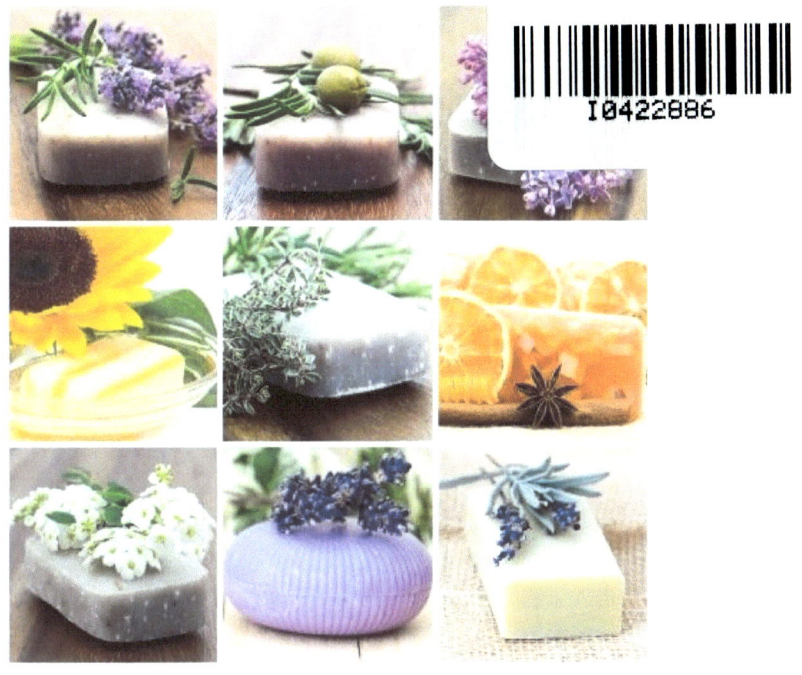

Elda Watulo

Health Learning Series
Mendon Cottage Books

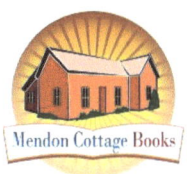

JD-Biz Publishing

Our books are available at

1. Amazon.com
2. Barnes and Noble
3. Itunes
4. Kobo
5. Smashwords
6. Google Play Books

Table of Contents

Introduction

Going green is all the rage right now, be it in fashion, in cars, in offices or what have you and why should you be left behind? In this book we look at the amazing natural products that are going to do wonders for your skin and hair as well as your general health. We look at the reasons why you cannot afford to continue using artificial beauty products and why it is about time you took a 360 degree turn on your current lifestyle.

This is a wellness book that holds important life lessons. Put your reading glasses on and let the journey that will change your life begin.

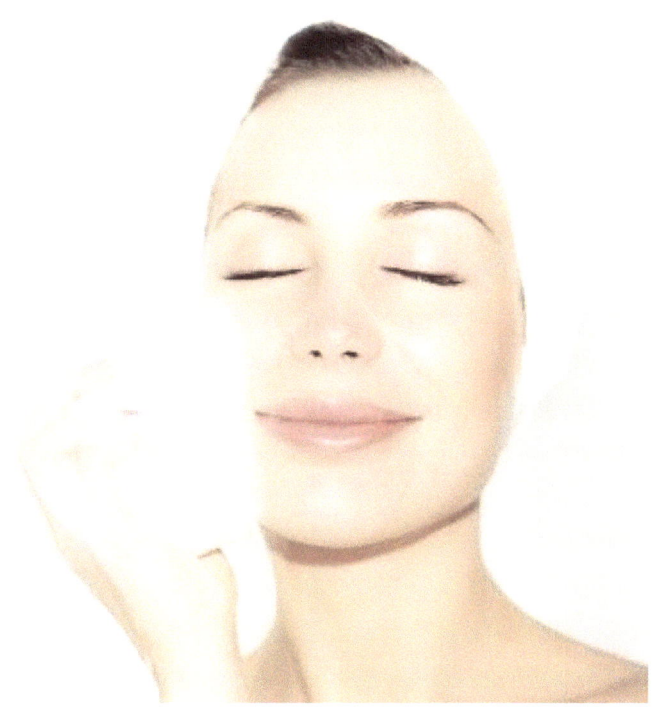

Chapter 1: The beauty of going natural

Our bodies are temples that need and deserve to be treated with the utmost care and love. Have you ever wondered why the ancient man had a body to die for? It is because they had no access to processed food and skin care products. They relied on Mother Nature for all their needs. Cancer and many other chronic diseases are at their all time high today and the reason if you ask me, is all the chemicals that we feed and expose our bodies to.

You may avoid cigarettes, alcohol, pesticides on fresh food and what have you but for as long as you are applying skin care products that are loaded with chemicals, you will in actual sense be doing zero work. There is no better time to go green on your body than now; from what you eat to what you breathe to what you apply on your skin and hair to everything that you interact with on a daily basis; you should completely steer away from anything that has chemicals as much as you can.

I am going to give you more reason for you to stop using processed health and beauty products by highlighting the benefits that you are going to accrue from going all natural.

Guard your body from chemicals

The skin is the body's largest organ and it consists of pores that readily absorb anything that is applied on the skin. It is common knowledge that 95% of beauty products contain a lot of chemicals and synthetic preservatives such as parabens, phthalates and petrochemicals that are supposed to give the product a longer shelf life. These chemicals can actually cause havoc in your body. These chemicals may at times mimic our natural hormones but the body does not respond to them in the same manner. Sometimes the body may identify them as aliens and launch an attack on them leading to very severe reactions like a breakout on your skin, nausea and constant headaches.

Again, as the chemicals keep getting absorbed little by little day by day in the end you may find yourself with a chronic disease that you might not understand its origin. To avoid all these, make a decision to throw away all your processed beauty products and start a new way of life by embracing the gifts of Mother Nature.

Sweet scents

Herbs, flowers, fruits and some seeds have essential oils that have the sweetest of scents. You cannot compare these to the chemical undertones used in artificial beauty products. To top it all, these essential oils also contain nutrients that do wonders for your skin and hair. Natural products are like a double edged sword; you get to have a beautiful scent and at the same time have silky smooth skin and hair courtesy of the nutrients in the products.

Economic sense

Natural health and beauty products are readily available right about everywhere in the whole world. If you go to your nearest drug store or supermarket, you are definitely going to find something like Epsom salt. You may not be familiar with this product but let me make you understand it. Epsom salt is a naturally occurring mineral that is made up of sulphate and magnesium. It is a very effective skin toner as well as exfoliate. In addition you can pour some Epsom salt in your bath water for a nice and relaxing bath.

Another amazing product is black cohosh which belongs to the buttercup flower family. It has a myriad of benefits some of which are reducing the harsh symptoms of menopause such as hot flushes and vaginal dryness.

Basically, there are so many naturally occurring products each with its own benefits that are very easy to acquire and at a very fair price. More often than not, artificial beauty products cost more than the natural products and if you consider the fact that you are always exposed to diseases such as cancer by using them; you are better off with the natural products.

Body friendly nutrients

Natural health and beauty products are made up of essential oils, vitamins, proteins and minerals that are very important for the normal function of the body. The fact that they are natural goes a long way in aiding the body to absorb them much faster as they are easily broken down unlike the artificial products that take a long time to get absorbed and what they are really doing is causing harm to the body.

Natural products also help in ridding the body of harmful toxins so every time you ingest or apply a natural product on your skin; you take a step further in cleansing yourself. If you are buying organic beauty products that are packaged, it is very important to check the labels to ensure that you are providing your skin with pure and natural products.

Save the world

There is so much pollution in our environment that the ozone layer is at a higher risk of getting depleted every passing day. The number one contributor of pollution is the refuse from artificial health and beauty products. Every single day as you take a bath and cleanse your face with artificial beauty products, chemicals go down your drain; when you spray yourself and your house with artificial products, again, chemicals are released in the air. So imagine millions and millions of people doing these every single day, how much pollution takes place?

We cannot reverse the effect of pollution but we can try and prevent any further pollution from taking place by using natural health and beauty products. In the first place, they are decomposable unlike the artificial beauty products.

These are the main benefits of using naturally occurring health and beauty products though the list is endless. One thing is for sure, if you and I treat our bodies like temples, we are going to be at our best health and our world is also going to be at its best health. A healthy world is most definitely a prosperous one. Let us join hands and improve the quality of life by going all natural.

Chapter 2: Fight diseases with natural products

You will be very amazed to discover that your pantry holds the key to a very healthy life. There are certain foods that are equipped with disease fighting nutrients. Once you discover this, you can say hello to a long and healthy life. We are going to look at nine super foods that have got effective disease fighting power.

Dairy products

Commonly known for their high level of calcium and protein, dairy is very rich in vitamin D and other minerals making it very good for combating Osteoporosis, a disease that affects the bones. Three servings of low fat dairy every day is all you need to stay away from Osteoporosis. Of course you also need to exercise for your bones to be nice, strong and healthy.

Alternative for lactose intolerant people and vegetarians

Calcium can also be found in dark leafy greens such as spinach, kale and broccoli; legumes such as beans, peas and green grams; juices and soy products that are calcium fortified.

Berries

Berries have got very high levels of antioxidants that are essential for neutralizing free radicals or in lay man's terms, cell damaging substances. This is very important for fighting chronic illnesses such as heart disease and cancer. Blue berries are at the very top of the list when it comes to high levels of antioxidants. Other berries rich in antioxidants are cranberries, blackberries, raspberries and strawberries. Anthocyanin is the antioxidant in berries that gives them their deep colors.

Cranberries are also known to fight off urinary tract infections. A cup of berries every single day is definitely going to go a long way in helping your body fight off these illnesses. You can put a spin to it by making a berry smoothie or using them as toppings in your frozen yoghurt or ice cream.

Tomatoes

Lycopene is an antioxidant found in ripe tomatoes that is very good in fighting and protecting against cancers. Additionally, they are rich in potassium, Vitamins A and C as well as phytochemicals. Tomatoes are readily available and can be eaten raw in salads or cooked. However way you like it; just ensure you eat at least two tomatoes a day.

Whole grains

Oatmeal is a staple in many kitchens for breakfast but what many people don't know is that the high fiber in oatmeal is very good for lowering blood cholesterol levels. Selenium, Folic acid and B vitamins are the essential nutrients that keep your heart healthy, reduce your risk of getting diabetes as well help you control your weight. All these wonderful nutrients are found in the component of whole grains that is usually stripped away when processing whole grains to get refined products. You will therefore be doing your body a disservice by feeding it with refined grain products.

You should at least take three servings of whole grain every day and they are so many; wild rice, quinoa, millet, oats, rye, brown rice, cereals, whole grain breads and pasta and so on.

Fish

The first thing that comes to mind when you hear of fish is Omega-3 fatty acids. As the name suggests, these are usually found in fatty fish such as salmon and tuna. Omega-3 fatty acids are great at lowering blood cholesterol as well as preventing blood clots that usually lead to cardiovascular diseases. Due to the high fat content, these fish should be eaten twice a week. Two servings of grilled tuna or salmon is definitely going to do so much for your heart.

Sweet potatoes

Phytochemicals such as beta-carotene, calcium, potassium, iron, copper, folate vitamins C and E are the nutrients contained in these orange tubers. Cancer and heart disease are the two diseases that are prevented every time you take sweet potatoes. In addition, they are rich in fiber that is great for promoting the health of your digestive tract.

Instead of taking white potatoes, take sweet potatoes and enjoy all these benefits. They are low fat so you will have no worries of adding a number of inches to your waist line.

Eggs

Eggs contain the carotenoids xeanthin, cholin and lutein and protein. They are very good for pregnant women and they also boost eye health as well as preventing macular degeneration that is associated with aging; this is usually the number one cause of blindness in the aged.

It is important to regulate your egg intake to avoid raising your cholesterol levels; you can take an egg every alternate day.

Legumes

If you include beans and other legumes regularly in your diet, you will significantly reduce your risk of getting cancer and you will also stabilize the sugar levels in your blood. Beans are loaded with iron, magnesium, folic acid, protein, fiber and phytochemicals. A good thing about legumes is that they are fat free and also very cheap and easy to get. They are also great if you are trying to shed some extra pounds as they keep you full for longer periods therefore keeping you from snacking all the time.

Nuts

Very rich in the healthy fats, also known as mono unsaturated fats, nuts are ideal for lowering cholesterol levels in the blood as well as fighting cardiovascular diseases. They are also rich in selenium, vitamins A and E, fiber and protein. Take a handful of nuts every single day for these health benefits. Remember to keep the portions small as they are high in calories and it is very easy for you to add weight if you overeat.

When you include all of the above foods in your diet, you can be sure never to see things like acne in your life; or if you are already suffering from acne, you can be sure to see a major improvement in your skin. When combined with water, this is going to have the best results for your body.

There are so many benefits to eating a healthy and natural diet but at least you can rest assured with these nine foods that you are going to wad off a number of diseases. By eating like this, you will have embraced the Paleolithic man's diet and you are definitely going to notice the difference in your skin, hair, weight as well as energy levels. You can never be too healthy for life, just steer away from artificial overly processed foods and load your fridge and pantry with these nine super foods.

Chapter 3: Natural products and allergies

There is nothing as uncomfortable as having an allergic reaction to something. You know that feeling, like an alien has taken over your body and there is nothing you can do about. Taking medication to stop these allergic reactions can also get cumbersome and that is why I am so excited to share with you some natural products that are definitely going to blow your mind.

Honey

Ever heard of the venom story where once you are bitten by a snake and treated of course, your immunity becomes stronger than before and if you are bitten a second time, the effects won't be as bad as the first time? Well, that is almost the same principle as honey. If you are allergic to pollen, licking natural honey is going to reduce these effects owing to the fact that honey is produced by bees which eat pollen. In essence, it is like taking an allergy shot.

Steam it up

A congested nose is one of the most common allergic reactions. One of the best and natural ways to combat this is to boil some water then add a few drops of eucalyptus oil, rosemary oil, tea tree oil, myrtle oil then place a towel over your head and inhale the steam for about 10 minutes. You will be breathing easily if you repeat this 2 more times.

Quercetin

This is naturally occurring in the skin of onions and is a great antihistamine. It is readily available in your local drug store and for an even stronger concoction, you can ask for a product that also contains bromelain, which is extracted from pineapples, another great antihistamine. You can seek for your doctor's advice on whether this is safe for you if in doubt.

Stinging nettle

The leaves of the stinging nettle can be used to make tea when combined with essential oils from rosemary and tea tree. This is a great combo for opening up a congested nose and chest.

Friendly bacteria

For those of us suffering from seasonal allergies, probiotics are a must. Acidophilus is a great probiotic that you should first get for preventive purposes. Additionally, probiotics boost the digestive system as well as the immune system. Visit your physician for the exact dosage that you should take.

Butterbur

This herbaceous perennial plant has got essential oils that contain sesquiterpenes that possess anti-inflammatory property. It is a great antihistamine and the best part is that it is naturally occurring. You can therefore switch your cetrizine bottle for this.

Vitamin C

The main cause of allergies is the histamine produced by our bodies when exposed to allergens. To combat this, you should increase your daily vitamin C intake and this will reduce the amount of histamine produced by your body. You will therefore have reduces instances of a runny nose or teary eyes.

Fish oils

EPA and DHA are the main components of essential fatty acids. These are very important in the process of the formation of each and every cell in the body. In addition to preventing heart disease, adding moisture to the skin and lowering cholesterol levels in the blood, they are good at combating hay fever. You cannot afford not have these in your diet for a generally healthy life.

Support your stress glands
Licorice is a great herb that does a very good job of reducing stress and increasing immunity. A regular intake of this herb is going to reduce the effect of allergies and stress in your body.

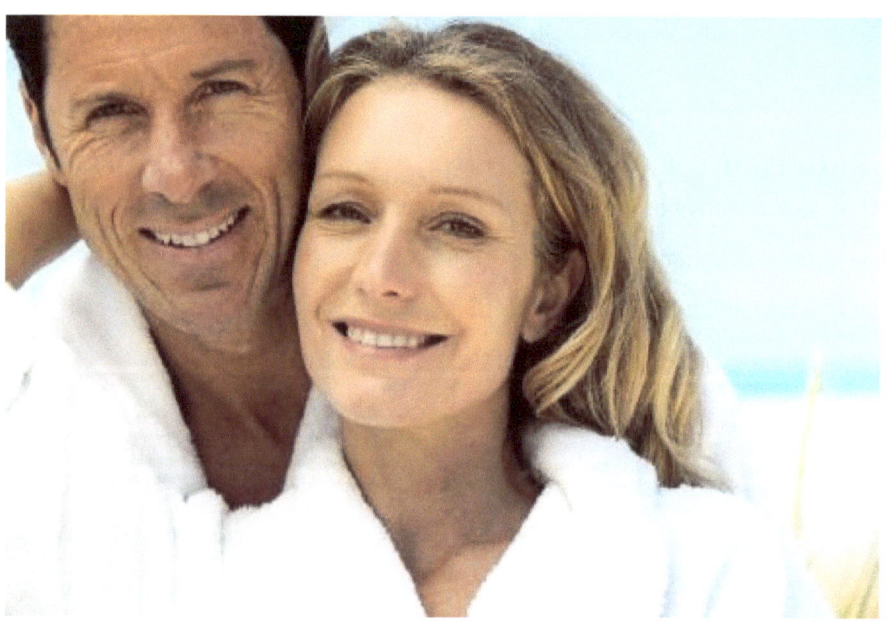

Mediterranean diet
This diet is very rich in fruits and veggies. It has been found to have a protective effect for kids with allergies and even asthma. It is very important to keep tabs on what goes into your diet especially during allergy season. Aim for a Mediterranean diet for increased immunity.

As we have seen, going natural is the best way to go for your health. Keep your allergies on check by following these simple guidelines and you will be a happier person but remember to avoid instances and places that are going to cause your allergies to flare up.

Chapter 4: Exercise caution with natural health and beauty products

Currently, natural health and beauty products are all the rage especially due to the fact that everyone seems to be embracing a healthier lifestyle and trying to stay cancer free. Celebrities in Hollywood and models alike are major campaigners of natural health and beauty products. Another thing that is making natural beauty products very popular is the belief that they are the answer to an even toned, smooth skin and long shiny hair among many other more benefits. It therefore comes as no surprise that everyone is going after these natural products.

Ideally, natural beauty products should contain little or no added chemicals making them perfect for our bodies. However, we need to be real; if you want nature in a bottle, then there has to be a bit of processing in the works. This is where you need to exercise a lot of caution because there are some unscrupulous people out there who are looking to make an easy dime by lying to people and making artificial products but labeling them as natural.

Some manufacturers may claim to use natural ingredients for their products only to find that they are using an imitation or flavoring instead of the real thing. The unfortunate part is that we do not have a clear regulation that distinctively defines how natural is natural and what products should or should not be used in making natural health and beauty products but hopefully this is soon going to change.

Learning to read labels is one thing that you need to do to avoid getting caught in the web of unethical manufacturers. Things you should be on the lookout for are; parabens, petrochemicals, mercury, lead, dioxane, and phthalates. These are very common in creams, lip balms, shampoos, mascara, nail polishes and foundations and are used to give beauty products a longer shelf life, as well as artificial scents.

One notion about natural beauty products is that they are purity in a bottle and therefore not capable of having any negative effects on your body. However, this is definitely not the case. Cases of allergies to some products are still there. You should especially be careful when using products containing lavender, tea tree oil and jasmine as there are cases of allergies to these that have been reported.

For people who are allergic to tree nuts, one should be very careful to avoid severe reactions that can at times be fatal. Read the label carefully to ensure that there is not even a strain of any tree nut. If you are not sure, you can ask your doctor if it is safe for you to use the product you are interested in.

Your nose can also be a great asset when it comes to identifying a true natural product from an imitation. If for example you are buying a strawberry lotion but instead it smells like a candy imitation, chances are that it is a fake natural body lotion.

At the end of the day, the decision lies with you. If you are ready to pay the extra price for the organic beauty product, well and good but you need to be privy to avoid getting short changed. Another thing is to know your body. Get to know what your skin type is so that at the end of the day you get a product that is definitely going to help you. In as much as you may have bought a natural product that is meant for a person with an oily skin; it will do nothing good to your dry skin.

You can also do a lot of research on a product that you are interested in. when you look at the products website or social media page you are sure to see reviews from people who have you used the product before. If the product is legit, you are going to see it from the positive comments. If more than 60% of the comments are negative, then obviously there is something wrong with the product.

If you ask me, if you your aim is to start using natural health and beauty products; go natural all the way. Instead of buying an organic shampoo, whip up something natural from your food in the kitchen. Stick to natural food products that have not been processed because either way, there is always an added chemical in processed products. Drink lots and lots of water and you are going to see a lot of positive changes in your body.

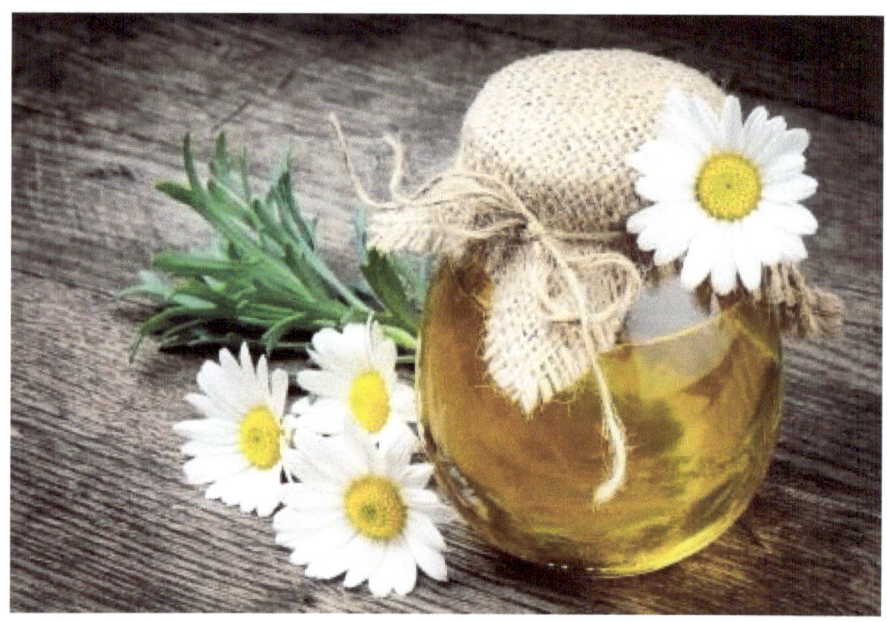

Chapter 5: Garbage in garbage out

When it comes to our appearances, no doubt we are always out to look our best; from how our skin and hair looks like to the clothes and shoes we wear; but there is one thing, you may have the best clothes and shoes that money can buy but if your skin and hair are not in their best shape, you will be left feeling like there is something missing.

Well, I have great news for you. There is away to polish up your look. You may already be using organic or natural beauty and health products but you need to go one step further; you need to feed your body with the right stuff.

It is true that garbage in equals garbage out. What this means is that whatever you put into your body is going to be reflected in your skin and hair as well as your eyes. You therefore need to start working from the inside out. Our aim is to stick to natural products as much as we can so things like candy bars and the like are an absolute no no.

Hydration is key in achieving inner and outer beauty. It is also a major component of natural beauty products as it is a natural moisturizer. Water also serves to flush out toxins from the body thereby leaving us with supple and healthy skin.

Fruits are another thing that should never miss from our diets. There are two things to this. You can ingest them as well as use them on your skin. Most natural beauty products manufacturers use lots and lots of fruits as their ingredients, they are loaded with vitamins and minerals that are key to a healthy body.

Foods that are rich in fiber are also very important. The moment your digestive system is in its best shape, you can be sure that your skin is also going to be in its best shape. You can therefore not afford to miss out on kale, spinach and the like.

Veggies are also loaded with iron and zinc that are very good for healthy hair as well as smooth skin. My advice would be to check out the various diets available such as the paleo diet and the Mediterranean diet; I am not talking about any crash diets. Borrow all the positive things from them and apply them to your own lifestyle.

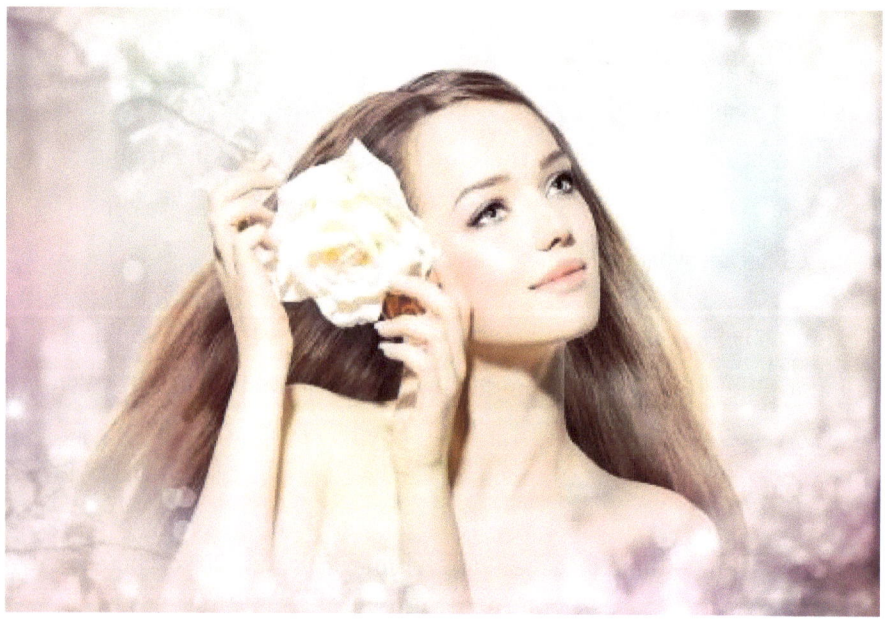

At the end of the day, it is a matter of saving you from cancer, heart disease and any other preventable disease by ensuring that you are not exposed to factors that your body was not designed to encounter. Again, we also need to save our environment. It will be of no use for us to be in the best health whilst our surroundings are in their worst possible shape.

Work from your inside to your outside; your attitude and outlook on life also count. Once you are happy with your inside, I can guarantee that your outside is also going to be perfect. Be natural, stay natural and do all things natural. There is no greater beauty than nature in itself. It is a great marvel and so should you be.

Chapter 6: Natural beauty products recipes

We are now going to look at a few recipes that are going to help you get that youthful glow on your skin as well as long luscious locks. My aim is to help you be in tip top shape in terms of beauty without having you break the bank. The best part is that you are going to use things that Are resting in your fridge and pantry and do not require a lot of work done.

Facial scrub

Ingredients

- ✓ 1 cup brown sugar
- ✓ 1 tsp real vanilla extract
- ✓ ¾ tsp vitamin E oil
- ✓ ¾ cup coconut oil
- ✓ 2 tbsps honey

Method

- Mix all the ingredients together and let them rest for 20 minutes apart from honey.
- Wet your face with a wash cloth then apply the mixture evenly on your face and neck. Rub gently until all the mixture falls off your face.
- Rinse your face with warm water then part it dry. Rub the honey on your face and leave it on for 20-30 minutes then rinse it off with warm water.
- Pat your face dry and apply 1-2 drops of coconut oil depending on your skin type

Sugar is definitely bad for your inner body but great for the skin. This is an amazing recipe that is all natural and that will leave your skin smooth and supple. Do this twice a week for the best results.

Lotion from the pantry
Ingredients

- ✓ 1 cup shea butter/ a=mango butter/ cocoa butter
- ✓ 1 cup beeswax
- ✓ 1 cup coconut oil
- ✓ 1/8 cup lavender essential oil (any other that you fancy)
- ✓ 1 ½ tsp vitamin E oil (for preservation)

Method

- Place some water in a sauce pan and bring to the boil. Mix all the ingredients in a glass bowl apart from the essential oil then place it over the boiling water.
- Stir constantly until the mixture completely melts.
- Remove the glass bowl from the boiling water and add the essential oil.
- Stir gently and when it's not too hot, use your hand until the essential oil is completely integrated with the rest of the mixture
- Pour the mixture into molds of desired shape and allow them to cool. Once they are completely cooled, pop them out and wrap them well.

You will definitely enjoy the silky smoothness of your skin with this recipe.

Wonder Shampoo
Ingredients

- ✓ ½ cup coconut milk
- ✓ ¾ cup liquid castile soap
- ✓ 2 tsps vitamin E oil
- ✓ 1/8 cup jasmine essential oil (any other essential oil of choice)
- ✓ 1 tsp olive oil, for people with a dry scalp

Method

- Take an old shampoo bottle and pour all the ingredients inside. Shake well until all the ingredients mix.
- Use this mixture for one month at most.

This is a healthy and aromatic way to clean your hair. Enjoy the fresh and cleaning courtesy of this wonder shampoo.

Soft hands

Ingredients

- ✓ 1 tbsp lemon juice
- ✓ 1tbsp honey
- ✓ 5 ground almonds
- ✓ 1 ½ tbsp sunflower oil
- ✓ 2 drops lavender essential oil

Method

- Mix all the ingredients until they form a thick paste.
- Let the mixture rest for about 15 minutes then apply it to your hands rubbing all the time. Leave it on for 10 minutes and rinse it off.

Walla! Say hi to your softer hands!

These are just a few of the products you can whip up in your kitchen. They are supposed to act as an eye opener for you so that you know the kind of ingredients you are supposed to use. Get creative and try a few things here and there and before you know it you will have discovered an amazing recipe for a lotion, perfume or even facial mask. One sure thing is that you are going to sleep better knowing that as each day passes, you are using less and less of processed beauty products and you are making your own from scratch.

Do a little research and shop for everything you need and get to work!

Conclusion

All along we have been looking at the importance of being natural and embracing nature as a whole, from what we put into our bodies as well as what we apply on our skin and our hair. This book is aimed at teaching you how to look after yourself and also the environment. We need to ensure that posterity has a place to call home. If we continue with our destructive ways of releasing chemicals into the environment; sooner rather than later we will not have earth to call home.

Embrace all these teachings and remember to take care of your body as it is your temple. No matter what anyone says, all natural is the way to go!

Author Bio

Elda Watulo is a Canada-based author of many award-winning books on different topics. She has published several health/fitness, business and marketing books, and she blogs at Hubpages.com.

Check out some of the other JD-Biz Publishing books

Health Learning Series

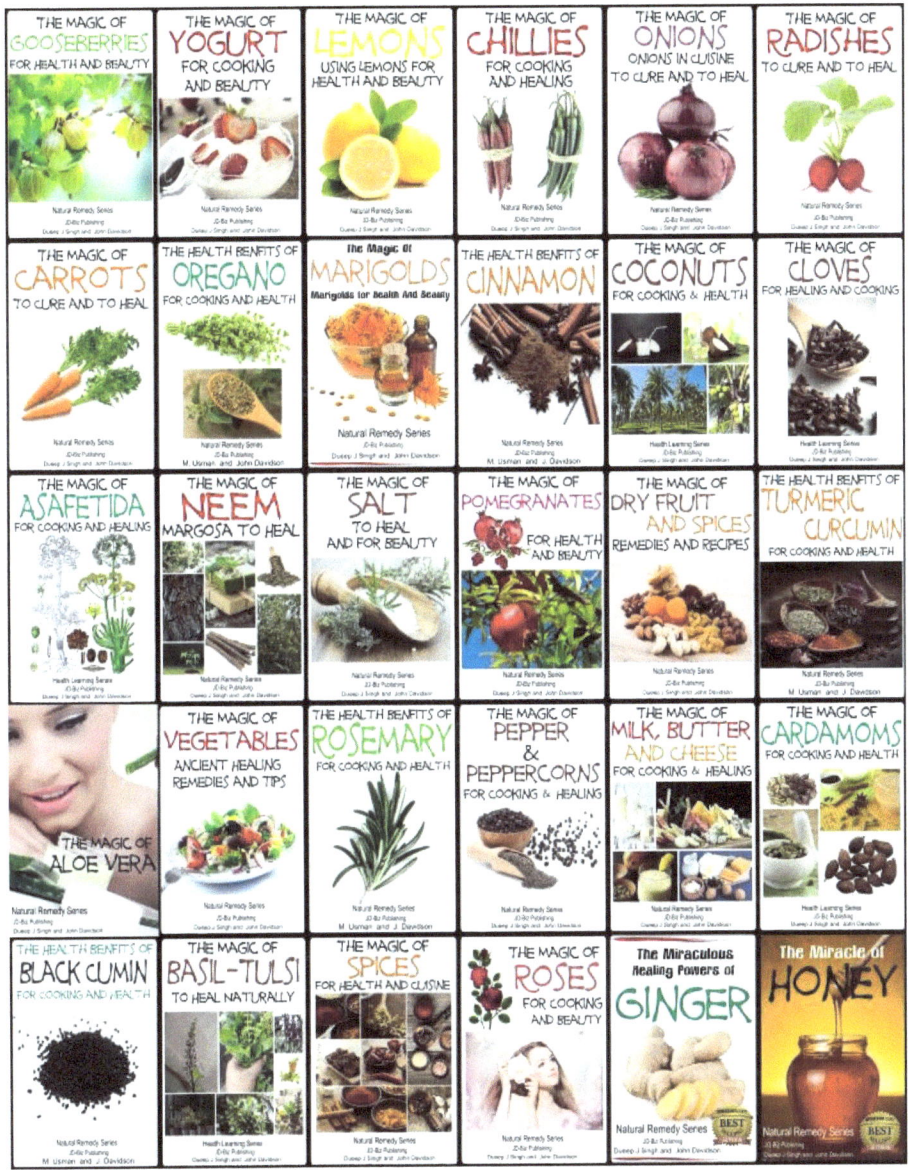

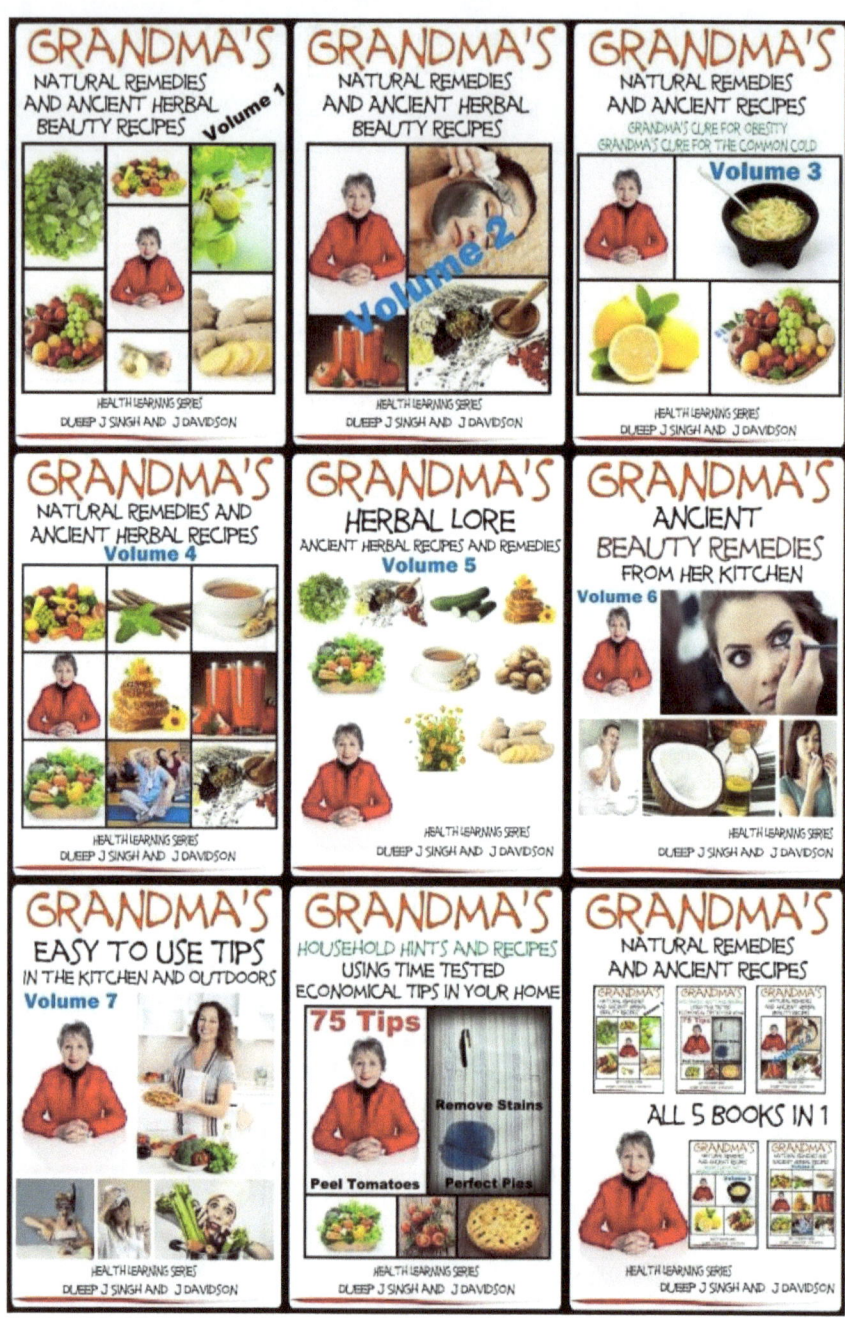

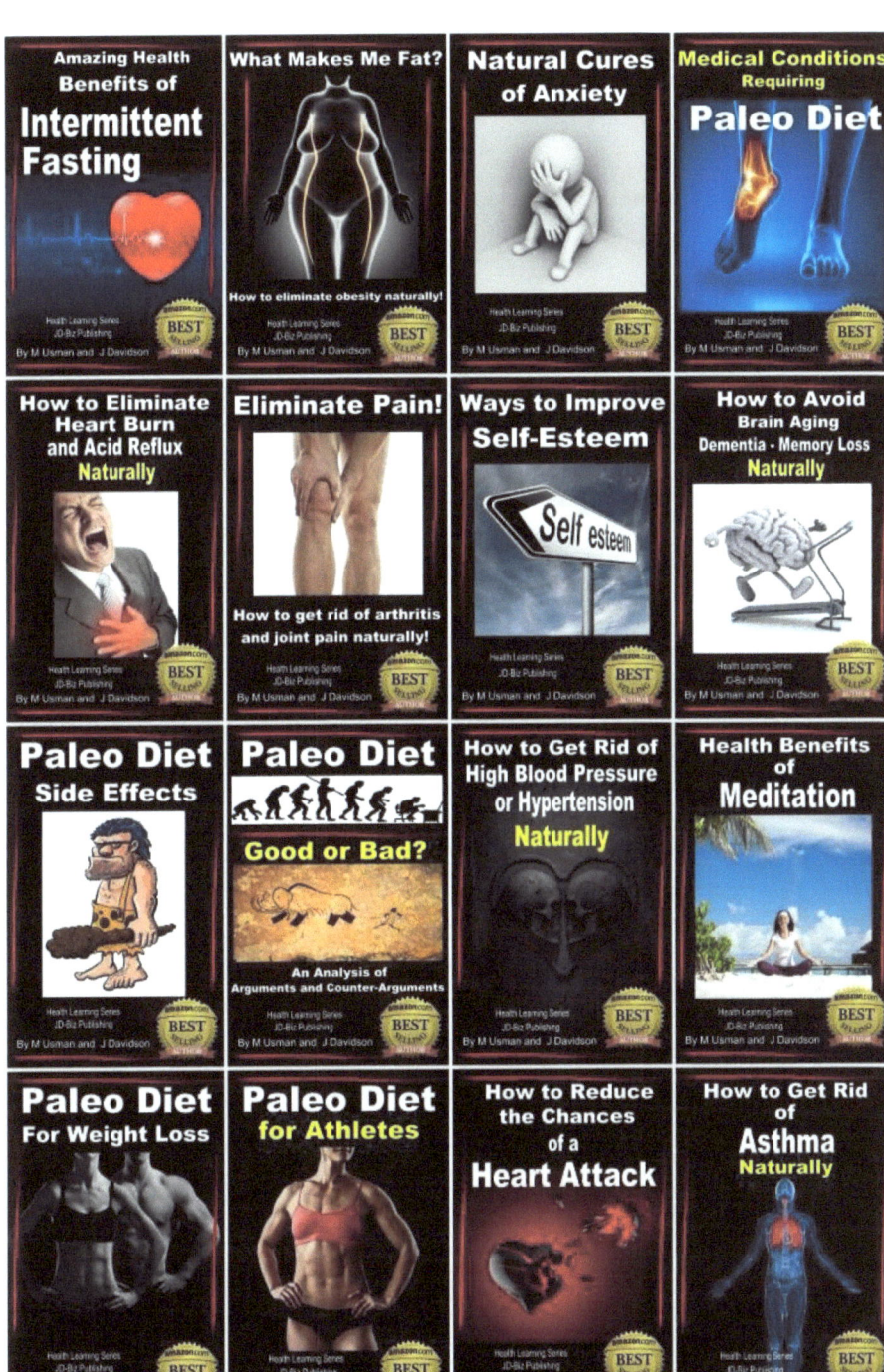

Amazing Animal Book Series

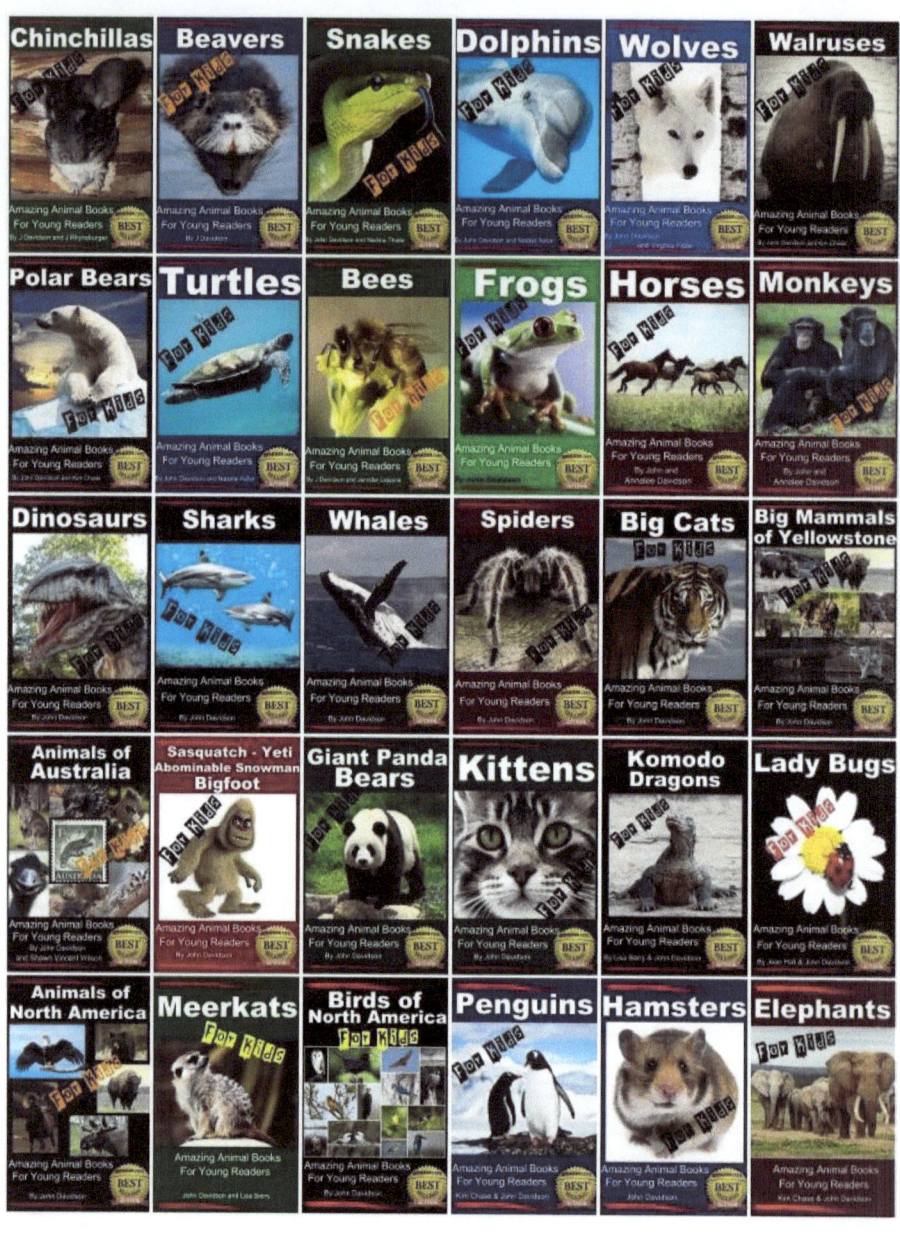

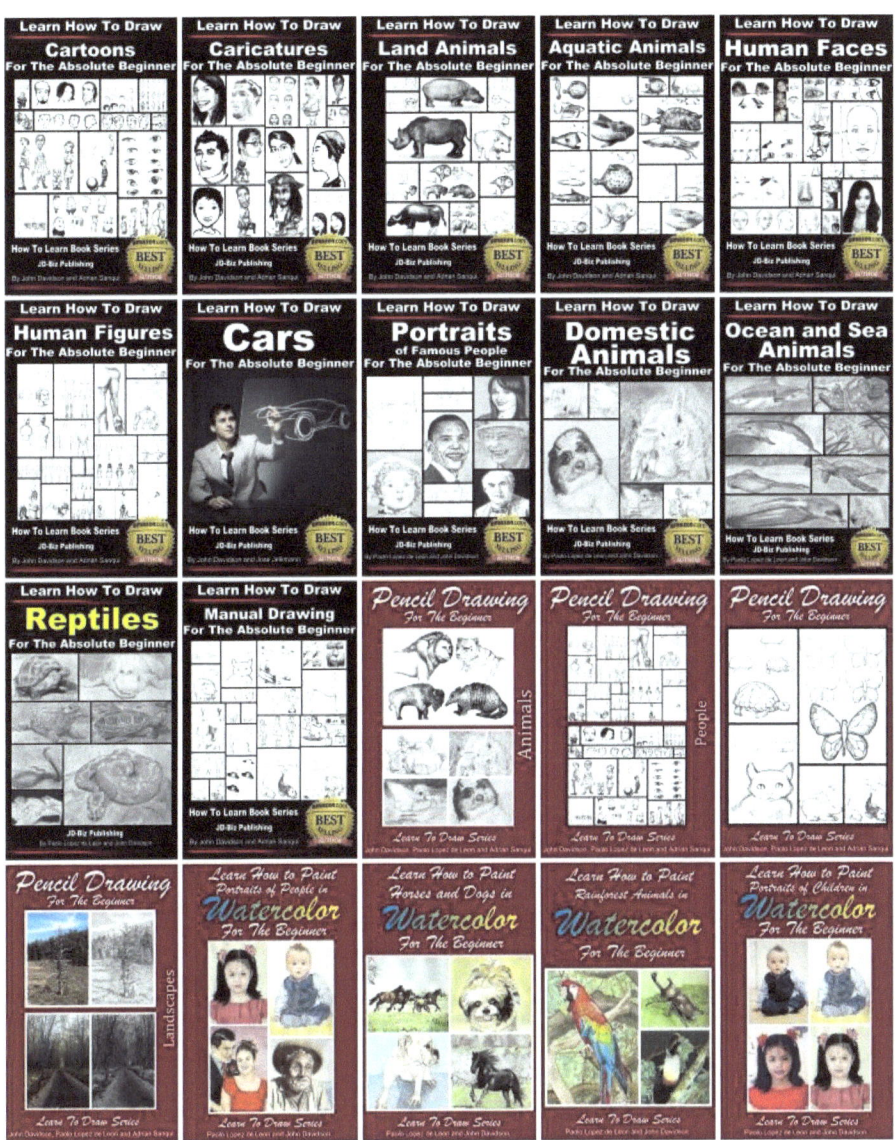

How to Build and Plan Books

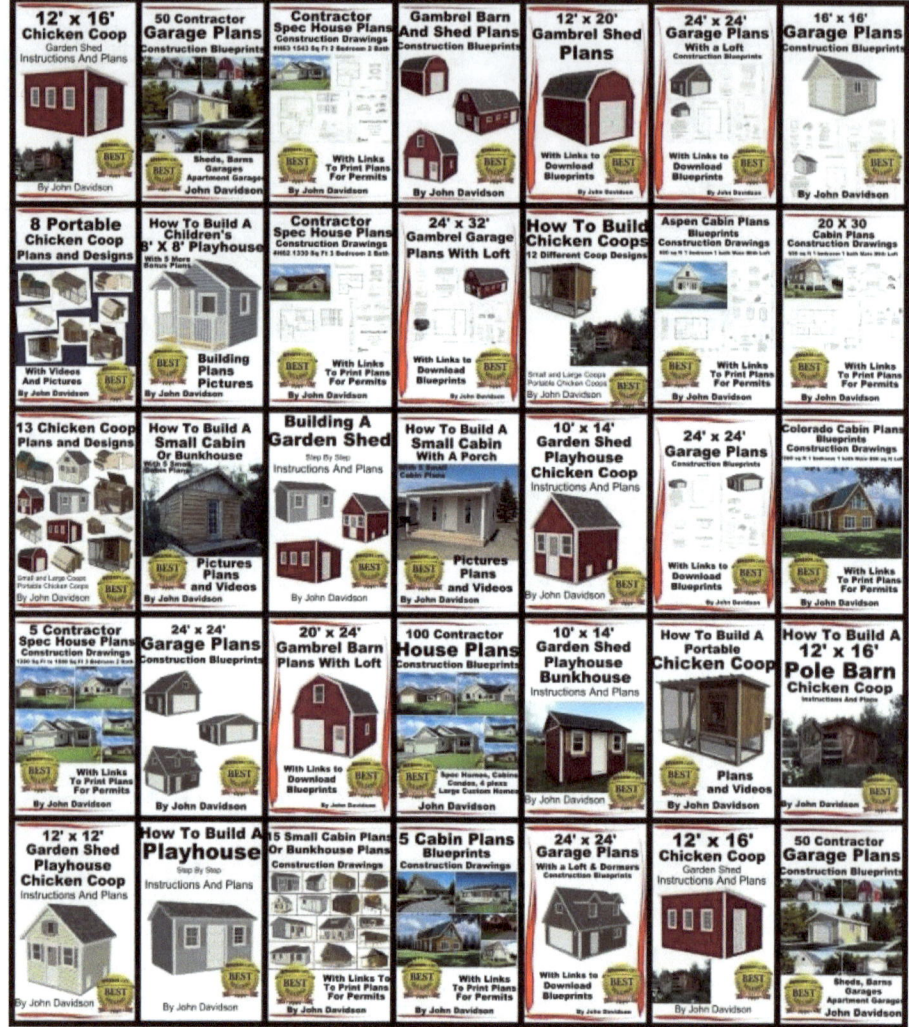

Entrepreneur Book Series

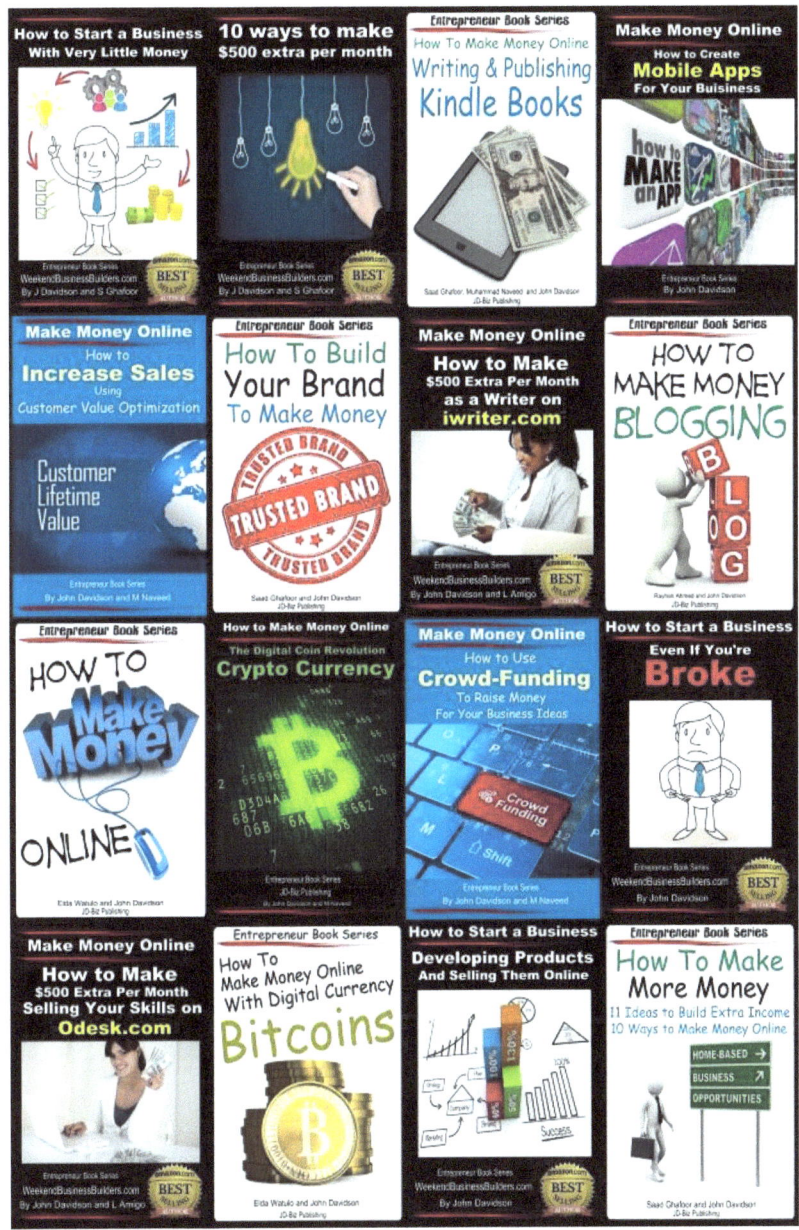

Our books are available at

1. Amazon.com

2. Barnes and Noble

3. Itunes

4. Kobo

5. Smashwords

6. Google Play Books

Download Free Books!

http://MendonCottageBooks.com

Publisher

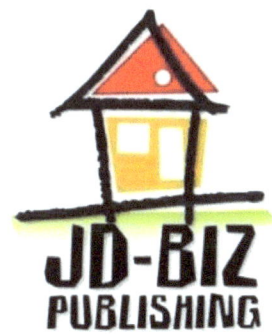

JD-Biz Corp

P O Box 374

Mendon, Utah 84325

http://www.jd-biz.com/

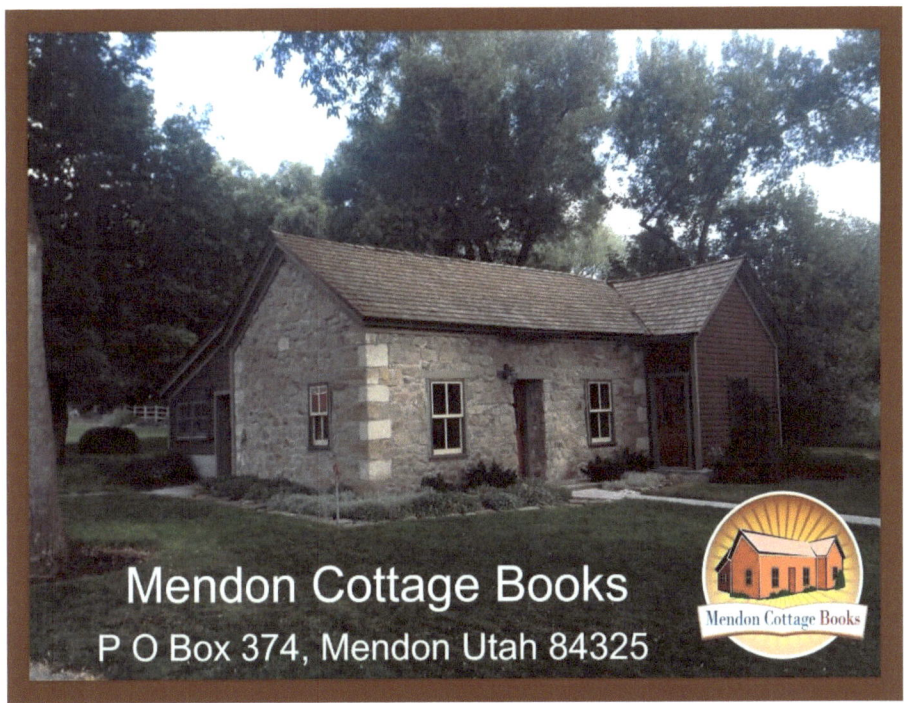

Mendon Cottage Books
P O Box 374, Mendon Utah 84325

www.ingramcontent.com/pod-product-compliance
Lightning Source LLC
Chambersburg PA
CBHW050903290526
45792CB00002B/683